Keto Chaffle Cookbook

Delicious, Easy, and Quick Low-Carb Waffle Recipes to Lose Weight and Share with Your Family Every Day.

Lucy Anderson

TABLE OF CONTENT

Introduction

Keto Chaffle is the latest and greatest invention in the keto world. This simple traditional Keto Chaffle recipe is a great bread substitute that works perfectly for making savory or sweet sandwiches.

Just like I'm not sure who invented the chaffle, I'm also not 100% sure where the name came from. The two main theories are these: is a combination of the words "cheese waffle" (which makes sense, especially when you see how it's made), or it is a combination of the words "chicken and waffle", which also makes sense because chicken and waffle have become very popular lately.

A chaffle is quite simple. It consists of only two ingredients: cheese and eggs. It's a cheese and egg waffle. It might not look too good at first, but trust me, it's really good!

Everyone is doing their chaffle so obviously, there is some variation. Some add yeast to make their chaffle get a little fluffier, while others simply add things like bacon to make it tastier. You can't go wrong.

If waffle-shaped grilled eggs and cheese aren't your things, don't worry, you can do it for yourself by adding whatever you want to the mix.

The texture of your chaffle

It takes four minutes to cook chaffle in a mini waffle maker. It will be soft and not very crunchy at first, but fear not! After you take the chaff out of the waffle maker and let it sit for a minute or two, it will start to get crunchy and give you a little crunch!

While the chaffle is amazing as it is, there are a few ways you might be able to make it even better. If you think your chaffle tastes too eggy, try using two egg whites instead of one whole egg. This seems to get rid of the egg.

While the chaffle is amazing as it is, there are a few ways you might be able to make it even better. If you think your chaffle tastes too eggy, try using two egg whites instead of one whole egg. This seems to get rid of the egg. Don't peek! I know it's tempting to want to see what's going on in your waffle maker, but if you open and close the machine while your chaffle is cooking, it will break and be a huge mess! Trust the process.

If you want your chaffle to be a little fluffier and have more texture, consider adding 1 teaspoon of baking powder to the batter or 1 tablespoon of almond flour. This will make your chaffle fresher.

If you have a family (or just love chaffles), consider purchasing a mini waffle maker that can make FOUR waffles at a time! Save time and effort and do all the cleaning you need all at once.

RECIPES

Garlic and Parsley Chaffle

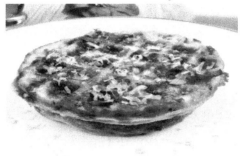

Preparation Time: 10 minutes **Cooking Time:** 5 Minutes

Servings:1

Ingredients:

- 1 large egg
- 1/4 cup cheese mozzarella
- 1 tsp. coconut flour
- ¼ tsp. baking powder
- ½ tsp. garlic powder
- 1 tbsp. minutes parsley

For Serving

- 1 Poach egg
- 4 oz. smoked salmon

Directions:

1. Switch on your Dash minutes waffle maker and let it preheat.
2. Grease waffle maker with cooking spray.
3. Mix together egg, mozzarella, coconut flour, baking powder, and garlic powder, parsley to a mixing bowl until combined well.
4. Pour batter in circle chaffle maker.
5. Close the lid.
6. Cook for about 2-3 minutes Utes or until the chaffles are cooked.
7. Serve with smoked salmon and poached egg.
8. Enjoy!

Nutrition:

Protein: 45% 140 kcal Fat: 51% 160 kcal Carbohydrates: 4% 14 kcal

Morning Chaffles With Berries

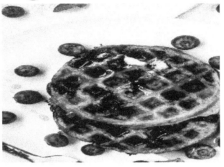

Preparation Time: 10 minutes **Cooking Time:** 5 Minutes

Servings: 4

Ingredients:

- 1 cup egg whites
- 1 cup cheddar cheese, shredded
- ¼ cup almond flour
- ¼ cup heavy cream

Topping

- 4 oz. raspberries
- 4 oz. strawberries.
- 1 oz. keto chocolate flakes
- 1 oz. feta cheese.

Directions:

1. Preheat your square waffle maker and grease with cooking spray.
2. Beat egg white in a small bowl with flour.
3. Add shredded cheese to the egg whites and flour mixture and mix well.
4. Add cream and cheese to the egg mixture.
5. Pour Chaffles batter in a waffle maker and close the lid.
6. Cook chaffles for about 4 minutes Utes until crispy and brown.
7. Carefully remove chaffles from the maker.
8. Serve with berries, cheese, and chocolate on top.
9. Enjoy!

Nutrition:

Protein: 28% 68 kcal Fat: 67% 163 kcal Carbohydrates: 5% 12 kcal

Keto Silver Dollar Pancakes

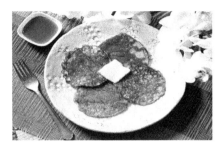

Preparation time: 10 minutes **Cooking time:** 5 minutes

Servings: 2

Ingredients:

- (3) Eggs
- 1/2 Cup (105 G) Cottage Cheese
- 1/3 Cup (37.33 G) Superfine Almond Flour
- 1/4 Cup (62.5 G) Unsweetened Almond Milk
- 2 Tablespoons Truvia
- Vanilla Extract
- 1 Teaspoon Baking Powder
- Cooking Oil Spray

Directions:

1. place ingredients in a blender in the order listed above. Mix until you have a smooth, fluid batter.

2. Heat a nonstick pan on medium-high temperature. Spray with oil or margarine.
3. Place 2 tablespoons of batter at once to make little, dollar hotcakes. This is an extremely fluid, sensitive batter so don't
4. attempt to make big pancakes with this one as they won't flip over easily.
5. Cooking every pancake until the top of the hotcake has made little air pockets and the air pockets have vanished, around 1-2 minutes.
6. Using a spatula, tenderly loosen the pan cake, and afterward flip over.
7. Make the remainder of the pancakes and serve hot.

Nutrition:

Calories: 110 Fat: 8g Protein: 2g Net Carbs: 7g

Chaffle Bowl

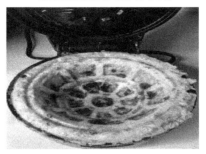

Preparation time: 10 minutes **Cooking time:** 5 minutes

Servings: 2

Ingredients:

- 1 Egg
- 1/2 cup cheddar cheese shredded pinch of Italian seasoning
- 1 tbsp. pizza sauce

Topping

- 1/2 Avocado Sliced
- 2 Eggs Boiled 1 Tomato, Halves
- 4 Oz. Fresh Spinach Leaves

Directions:

1. Preheat your waffle maker and grease with cooking

spray.

2. Crack an egg in a small bowl and beat with Italian seasoning and pizza sauce.

3. Add shredded cheese to the egg and spices mixture. Pour 1 tbsp. shredded cheese in a waffle maker and cooking for 30 sec.

4. Pour Chaffles batter in the waffle maker and close the lid.

5. Cooking chaffles for about 4 minutes until crispy and brown. Carefully remove chaffles from the maker.

6. Serve on the bed of spinach with boil egg, avocado slice, and tomatoes. Enjoy!

Nutrition:

Calories: 75 Fat: 6g Protein: 2.5g Net Carbs: 2g

Delicious Raspberries Chaffles

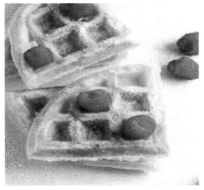

Preparation time: 20 minutes **Cooking time:** 15 minutes

Servings: 1

Ingredients:

- 1 egg white
- 1/4 cup jack cheese, shredded
- 1/4 cup cheddar cheese, shredded
- 1 tsp. coconut flour
- 1/4 tsp. baking powder
- 1/2 tsp. stevia
- For Topping
- 4 oz. raspberries
- 2 tbsps. coconut flour
- 2 oz. unsweetened raspberry sauce

Directions:

1. Switch on your round Waffle Maker and grease it with cooking spray once it is hot.
2. Mix together all chaffle ingredients in a bowl and combine with a fork. 3. Pour chaffle batter in a preheated maker and close the lid.
3. Roll the taco chaffle around using a kitchen roller, set it aside and allow it to set for a few minutes.
4. Once the taco chaffle is set, remove from the roller.
5. Dip raspberries in sauce and arrange on taco chaffle.
6. Drizzle coconut flour on top.
7. Enjoy raspberries taco chaffle with keto coffee.

Nutrition:

Calorie Count: 54 Protein: 3 g Fat: 4.1 g Carbohydrates: 1.1 g

Japanese Chaffle

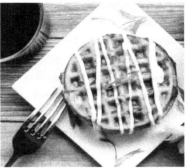

Preparation time: 12 minutes **Cooking time:** 6 minutes

Servings: 2

Ingredients:

- Egg: 1
- Bacon: 1 slice
- Green onion: 1 stalk
- Mozzarella cheese: 1/2 cup (shredded)
- Kewpie Mayo: 2 tablespoons

Directions:

1. Preheat and grease the waffle maker. Using a mixing bowl, a mix containing kewpie mayo with beaten egg, then add in ½ chopped green onion with the other ½ kept aside, and ¼ inches of cut bacon into the mixture.
2. Mix evenly. Sprinkle the base of the waffle maker with

21

1/8 cup of shredded Mozzarella and pour in the mixture, then top with more shredded mozzarella. With a closed lid, heat the waffle for 5 minutes to a crunch and then remove the chaffle and allow cooking for a few minutes. Repeat for the remaining chaffles mixture to make more batter.

3. Serve by garnishing the chaffle with the leftover chopped green onions. Enjoy.

Nutrition:

Calories 92 Kcal Fat: 7 g Protein: 1 g Net carb: 2 g

Keto Chaffle Bacon Sandwich

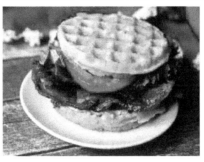

Preparation time: 15 minutes **Cooking time:** 10 minutes

Servings: 2

Ingredients:

- 1 egg ½ cup of shredded Mozzarella cheese
- 2 Tablespoon of coconut flour
- 2 strips of pork or beef bacon
- 1 slice of any type of cheese
- 2 tablespoon of coconut oil

Directions:

1. To make the chaffle, you will be following the typical recipe for making a chaffle. Start by warming your waffle machine to medium heat. In a bowl, beat 1 egg, ½ cup of Mozzarella cheese, and almond flour. Pour the mixture on the waffle machine. Let it cooking until it is

golden brown. Then remove in a plate.

2. Warm coconut oil in a pan over medium heat. Then place the bacon strips in the pan.

3. Cooking until crispy over medium heat. Assemble the bacon and cheese on the chaffle.

Nutrition:

Calories: 225 Fat: 19g Protein: 8g Net Carbs: 3g

Pork Chaffles

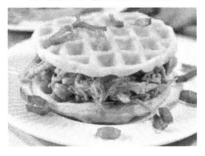

Preparation time: 10 minutes **Cooking time:** 10 minutes

Servings: 4

Ingredients:

- cup pulled pork, cooked
- 2 tablespoons parmesan, grated
- 2 eggs, whisked 2 red chilies, minced
- 1 cup almond milk
- 1 cup almond flour
- 2 tablespoons coconut oil, melted
- 1 teaspoon baking powder

Directions:

1. In a bowl, mix the pulled pork with the eggs, parmesan and the other ingredients and whisk well.
2. Heat up the waffle maker, pour ¼ of the chaffle mix,

cooking for 8 minutes and transfer to a plate.

3. Repeat with the rest of the mix and serve.

Nutrition:

Net Carbs: 0.1g; Calories: 110.7; Total Fat: 8g; Saturated Fat: 1.2g; Protein: 9.4g; Carbs: 0.3g; Fiber: 0.2g; Sugar: 0.2g

Hot Pesto Chaffles

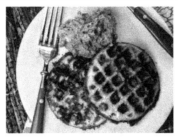

Preparation time: 10 minutes **Cooking time:** 7 minutes

Servings: 4

Ingredients:

- 1 cup almond milk
- 1 cup mozzarella, shredded
- 1 cup coconut flour
- 3 tablespoons basil pesto
- 1 teaspoon hot paprika
- 1 teaspoon chili powder
- 2 eggs, whisked
- 1 tablespoon ghee, melted
- 1 teaspoon baking soda

Directions:

1. In a bowl, mix the milk with the cheese, pesto and the other ingredients and whisk.

2. Heat up the waffle maker, pour ¼ of the mix, cooking for 7 minutes and transfer to a plate.

3. Repeat with the rest of the mix and serve.

Nutrition:

Calories 101 Fat 7.4g Fiber 3.2g Carbs 8.3g Protein 3.1g

BBQ Chicken Chaffle Sandwich

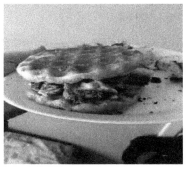

Preparation time: 10 minutes **Cooking time:** 7 minutes

Servings: 4

Ingredients:

- Boneless chicken breast 2 pieces
- BBQ Sauce (sugar-free)
- ¼ tsp. paprika
- 1 tablespoon lime juice
- ¼ tsp. of salt ¼ tsp. of pepper
- 1 piece of coal ½ cup of cheddar cheese
- 1 egg
- ½ tablespoon of Italian herbs
- 1 slice of cheese
- ½ tomato (sliced)
- 2 slices of lettuce
- ½ tablespoon oil

Directions:

1. To make your BBQ chicken chaffle sandwich, start by the preparation of your chicken. Take the boneless chicken pieces and cut them into cubes. Then marinate the cubes with Italian herbs, paprika, lime juice, oil, salt, and pepper. Then mix them thoroughly. Let the marination set on the chicken for around 20 minutes.

2. Then melt the butter in a pan and cooking your chicken in it.

3. Take the piece of coal and burn it. Use a tong to pick it up and place it in an aluminum foil. Put the coal on the chicken and cover it with a lid.

4. Let the chicken cooking with the smoky flavor for around 7 to 10 minutes. Then remove the chicken and place it in a dish. Then start preparing your chaffle bread. Preparing the chaffle bread is easy and requires only two ingredients. Whisk together egg and cheddar cheese.

5. You can add some Italian seasonings to give some taste to the bread. Then preheat your waffle maker to medium heat and pour the mixture into the machine.

6. Cooking it well for about 3 to 5 minutes. Repeat the process to get another chaffle.

7. Then assemble your sandwich. Put the chicken into the

chaffle bread and add tomatoes, lettuce, BBQ sauce, and a cheese slice to your sandwich. Voila! Your keto sandwich is ready.

Nutrition:

Calories 158 Fat 13.3g Fiber 3.9g Carbs 8.9g Protein 3.3g

Simple & Savory Chaffle

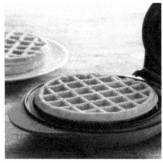

Preparation time: 10 minutes **Cooking time:** 10 minutes

Servings: 4

Ingredients:

- Batter
- 4 eggs
- 1 cup grated mozzarella cheese
- 1 cup grated provolone cheese
- ½ cup almond flour 2 tablespoons coconut flour
- 2½ teaspoons baking powder
- Salt and pepper to taste Other
- 2 tablespoons butter to brush the waffle maker

Directions:

1. Preheat the waffle maker.
2. Add the grated mozzarella and provolone cheese to a

bowl and mix.

3. Add the almond and coconut flour and baking powder and season with salt and pepper.

4. Mix with a wire whisk and crack in the eggs.

5. Stir everything together until batter forms.

6. Brush the heated waffle maker with butter and add a few tablespoons of the batter.

7. Close the lid and cook for about 8 minutes depending on your waffle maker.

8. Serve and enjoy.

Nutrition:

Calories 352, fat 27.2 g, carbs 8.3 g, sugar 0.5 g, Protein 15 g, sodium 442 mg

Gruyere and Chives Chaffles

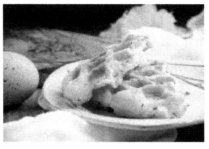

Preparation time: 15 minutes **Cooking time:** 15 minutes

Servings: 2

Ingredients:

- 2 eggs, beaten
- 1 cup finely grated Gruyere cheese
- 2 tbsp finely grated cheddar cheese
- 1/8 tsp freshly ground black pepper
- 3 tbsp minced fresh chives + more for garnishing
- 2 sunshine fried eggs for topping

Directions:

1. Preheat the waffle iron.
2. In a medium bowl, mix the eggs, cheeses, black pepper, and chives.
3. Open the iron and pour in half of the mixture.
4. Close the iron and cook until brown and crispy, 7

minutes.

5. Remove the chaffle onto a plate and set aside.

6. Make another chaffle using the remaining mixture.

7. Top each chaffle with one fried egg each, garnish with the chives and serve.

Nutrition:

Calories: 99 Cal Total Fat: 8 g Saturated Fat: 0 g Cholesterol: 0 mg Sodium: 0 mg Total Carbs: 4 g

Keto Chaffle Waffle

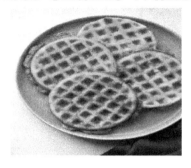

Preparation time: 15 minutes **Cooking time:** 10 minutes

Servings: 2

Ingredients:

- 1 egg
- ½ cup of shredded Mozzarella cheese
- 1 ½ table-spoon of almond flour
- Pinch of baking powder

Directions:

1. Start by turning your waffle maker on and preheating it. During the time of pre-heating, in a bowl, whisk the egg and shredded Mozzarella cheese together. If you do not have shredded Mozzarella cheese, you can use the shredder to shred your cheese, then add the almond powder and baking powder to the bowl and whisk them

until the mixture is consistent.

2. Then pour the mixture onto the waffle machine. Make sure you pour it to the center of the mixture will come out of the edges on closing the machine.

3. Close the machine and let the waffles cooking until golden brown. Then you can serve your tasty chaffle waffles.

Nutrition:

Calories: 170 Fat: 15g Protein: 7g Net Carbs: 2g

Lemon Almonds Chaffle

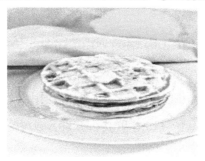

Preparation time: 15 minutes **Cooking time:** 10 minutes

Servings: 2

Ingredients:

- Cheddar cheese: 1/3 cup
- Egg: 1
- Lemon juice: 2 tbsp.
- Almond flour: 2 tbsp.
- Baking powder: 1/4 teaspoon
- Ground almonds: 2 tbsp.
- Mozzarella cheese: 1/3 cup

Directions:

1. Mix cheddar cheese, egg, lemon juice, almond flour, almond ground, and baking powder together in a bowl.
2. Preheat your waffle iron and grease it.

3. In your mini waffle iron, shred half of the Mozzarella cheese.
4. Add the mixture to your mini waffle iron.
5. Again, shred the remaining Mozzarella cheese on the mixture.
6. Cooking till the desired crisp is achieved.
7. Make as many chaffles as your mixture and waffle maker allow.

Nutrition:

Calories: 594 kcal Protein: 38.45 g Fat: 44.5 g Carbohydrates: 11.71 g Sodium: 914 mg

Peanut Butter Cup Chaffles

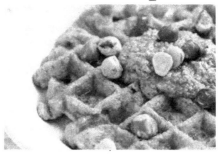

Preparation time: 5 minutes **Cooking time:** 15 minutes

Servings: 1

Ingredients:

For the chaffle:

- Eggs: 1
- Mozzarella cheese: ½ cup shredded
- Cocoa powder: 2 tbsp.
- Espresso powder: ¼ tsp.
- Sugar free chocolate chips: 1 tbsp.

For the filling:

- Peanut butter: 3 tbsp.
- Butter: 1 tbsp.
- Powdered sweetener: 2 tbsp.

Directions:

1. Add all the chaffle ingredients in a bowl and whisk.
2. Preheat your mini waffle iron if needed and grease it.
3. Cooking your mixture in the mini waffle iron for at least 4 minutes. Make two chaffles
4. Mix the filling ingredients together.
5. When chaffles cool down, spread peanut butter on them to make a sandwich.

Nutrition:

Calories: 448; Total Fat: 34g; Carbs: 17g; Net Carbs: 10g; Fiber: 7g; Protein: 24g

Chaffles With Egg & Asparagus

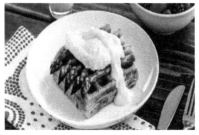

Preparation time: 15 minutes **Cooking time:** 10 minutes

Servings: 1

Ingredients:

- 1 egg
- 1/4 cup cheddar cheese
- 2 tbsps. almond flour
- ½ tsp. baking powder
- Topping
- 1 egg 4-5 stalks asparagus
- 1 tsp avocado oil

Directions:

1. Preheat waffle maker to medium-high heat.
2. Whisk together egg, mozzarella cheese, almond flour, and baking powder Pour chaffles mixture into the center of the waffle iron. Close the waffle maker and let

cook for 5 minutes Utes or until waffle is golden brown and set.

3. Remove chaffles from the waffle maker and serve.
4. Meanwhile, heat oil in a nonstick pan.
5. Once the pan is hot, fry asparagus for about 4-5 minutes Utes until golden brown.
6. Poach the egg in boil water for about 2-3 minutes Utes.
7. Once chaffles are cooked, remove from the maker.
8. Serve chaffles with the poached egg and asparagus.

Nutrition:

Calories: 843 Total Fat: 65g Saturated Fat: 14g Protein: 59g Cholesterol: 156mg Carbohydrates: 6g Fiber: 1g Net Carbs: 5g

Chocolate Chaffles

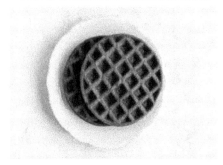

Preparation time: 5 minutes **Cooking time:** 15 minutes

Servings: 1

Ingredients:

- ggs: 1
- Mozzarella cheese: ½ cup shredded
- Cocoa powder: 2 tbsp.
- Espresso powder: ¼ tsp.
- Sugar free chocolate chips: 1 tbsp.

Directions:

1. Add all the chaffle ingredients in a bowl and whisk.
2. Preheat your mini waffle iron if needed and grease it.
3. Cooking your mixture in the mini waffle iron for at least 4 minutes. Make as many chaffles as you can.

Nutrition:

Calories: 258; Total Fat: 23g; Carbs: 12g; Net Carbs: 6g; Fiber: 6g; Protein: 5g

Zucchini and Onion Chaffles

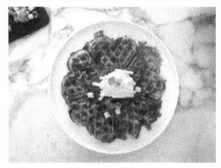

Preparation time: 15 minutes **Cooking time:** 15 minutes

Servings: 2

Ingredients:

- 2 cups zucchini, grated and squeezed
- ½ cup onion, grated and squeezed
- 2 organic eggs
- ½ cup Mozzarella cheese, shredded
- ½ cup Parmesan cheese, grated

Directions:

1. Preheat a waffle iron and then grease it.
2. In a medium bowl, place all ingredients and, mix until well combined. Place ¼ of the mixture into preheated waffle iron and cook for about 4 minutes or until golden brown.

3. Repeat with the remaining mixture. Serve warm.

Nutrition:

Net Carbs: 2g; Calories: 193.6; Total Fat: 12g; Saturated Fat: 1.7g; Protein: 17g; Carbs: 5g; Fiber: 3g; Sugar: 2.5g

Keto Cauliflower Chaffles Recipe

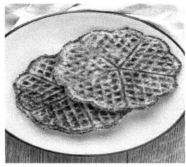

Preparation time: 1 minutes **Cooking time:** 5 minutes

Servings: 2

Ingredients:

- 1 cup of cauliflower, riced
- 1/4 tsp. of garlic powder
- 1/4 tsp. of black pepper, ground
- 1/2 tsp. of Italian Seasoning
- 1/4 tsp. of Kosher salt
- 1/2 cup of Mozzarella cheese shredded
- 1 egg
- 1/2 cup of parmesan cheese, shredded

Directions:

1. Combine all the ingredients and put them into a blender.

2. In waffle maker, scatter 1/8 cup of parmesan cheese. Ensure the waffle iron bottom is covered.

3. Pour the cauliflower batter into the waffle machine.

4. Put another scattering of parmesan cheese on the mixture's top. Ensure the top of the waffle iron is covered.

5. Cooking it for 4 to 5 min, or till its crispy.

6. Tends to make four mini chaffles or two full-size chaffles.

Nutrition:

Calories: 265 Net Carbs: 0 g Fat: 9 g Protein: 8 g

Japanese Style Chaffle Pizza

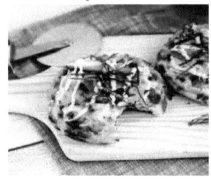

Preparation time: 12 minutes **Cooking time:** 5 minutes

Servings: 2

Ingredients:

- Mozzarella cheese: 1 cup (shredded)
- Egg: 2

Toppings

- Pizza sauce: 4 tablespoons
- Japanese sausage: 2 wholes
- Asparagus: 2 stalks
- Mozzarella cheese: 2 tablespoons (shredded)
- Kewpie mayo: 2 tablespoons
- Dried seaweed: 2 teaspoons

Directions:

1. Quickly, preheat a mini-sized waffle and grease it.
2. Using a mixing bowl, a mixture containing beaten eggs with Mozzarella cheese, mix evenly and pour into the lower side of the waffle maker.
3. With close lid, cool for 5 minutes to a crunch.
4. Preheat an oven to 500F, with the chaffle on a baking tray, pizza topping by adding the Asparagus and Japanese sausage into ¼ inch.
5. Spread the sliced asparagus, Japanese sausage and kewpie mayo on the pizza sauce on the chaffle.
6. Bake in the oven for 4 minutes at 500F until cheese melts.
7. Garnish on the top with shredded dried seaweed and enjoy.

Nutrition:

Calories: 41 Net Carbs: 0.3 g Fat: 35.2 gProtein: 26.7 g

Vegetable Pizza Chaffle

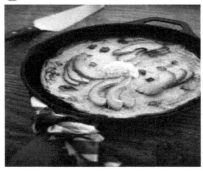

Preparation time: 20 minutes **Cooking time:** 25 minutes

Servings: 2

Ingredients:

Topping

- Tomato sauce: 2 teaspoons (sugar-free)
- Cauliflower: 4 tablespoons (diced)
- Mozzarella cheese: ½ cup shredded
- Onion: 4 tablespoons (diced)
- Olives: 4 tablespoons (diced)
- Red pepper: 4 tablespoons (diced)
- Tomatoes: 4 tablespoons (diced)
- Butter: 1 tablespoon
- Salt: a pinch

Pizza Chaffles

- Eggs: 2
- Italian season: ¼ teaspoon
- Cheddar cheese: ½ cup
- Parmesan cheese: 2 tablespoons

Directions:

1. Heat some butter in a saucepan with the vegetables (onion, tomatoes, cauliflower, red pepper) and salt for 3 minutes and keep aside.
2. Preheat and grease a waffle maker. a combined mixture of all Pizza chaffles ingredients, evenly mixed and pour into the base of waffle maker evenly and spread.
3. With closed lids, cooking for 4 minutes till chaffles turn crispy, and then set aside.
4. Transfer the chaffle into a parchment paper-lined up.
5. Pour some tomato sauce with the vegetable mixture on each chaffle and sprinkle with shredded Mozzarella cheese.
6. Bake the chaffle in the oven for 2 minutes until the cheese turns light brown.
7. The dish is ready.

Nutrition:

Calories 338 Total Fat 3.8 g Saturated Fat 0.7 g Cholesterol 22 mg Total Carbs 8.3 g Fiber 2.4 g Sugar 1.2 g Sodium 620 mg Potassium 271 mg Protein 15.4g

Chicken Chaffle

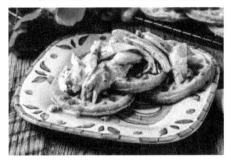

Preparation time: 10 minutes **Cooking time:** 15 minutes

Servings: 2

Ingredients:

- 2 oz chicken breasts, cooked, shredded
- 1/2 cup mozzarella cheese, finely shredded
- 2 eggs
- 6 tbsp parmesan cheese, finely shredded
- 1 cup zucchini, grated
- ½ cup almond flour
- 1tsp baking powder
- ¼ tsp garlic powder
- ¼ tsp black pepper, ground
- ½ tsp Italian seasoning
- ¼ tsp salt

Directions:

1. Sprinkle the zucchini with a pinch of salt and set it aside for a few minutes. Squeeze out the excess water.
2. Warm up your mini waffle maker.
3. Mix chicken, almond flour, baking powder, cheeses, garlic powder, salt, pepper and seasonings in a bowl.
4. Use another small bow for beating eggs. Add them to squeezed zucchini, mix well.
5. Combine the chicken and egg mixture, and mix.
6. For a crispy crust, add a teaspoon of shredded cheese to the waffle maker and cook for 30 seconds.
7. Then, pour the mixture into the waffle maker and cook for 5 minutes or until crispy.
8. Carefully remove. Repeat with remaining batter the same steps.

Nutrition:

Calories: 341 Total Fat: 27g Protein: 21g Total Carbs: 1g Fiber: 0g Net Carbs: 1g Cholesterol: 134mg

Chaffle Sandwich

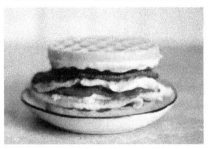

Preparation time: 20 minutes **Cooking time:** 15 minutes

Servings: 2

Ingredients:

- Cooking spray
- 4 slices bacon
- 1 tablespoon mayonnaise
- 4 basic chaffles
- 2 lettuce leaves
- 2 tomato slices

Directions:

1. Coat your pan with foil and place it over medium heat. Cooking the bacon until golden and crispy.
2. Spread mayo on top of the chaffle.
3. Top with the lettuce, bacon and tomato.
4. Top with another chaffle.

Nutrition:

Kcal 398, Fat 32g, Net Carbs 4g, Protein 24g

Walnuts Chaffles

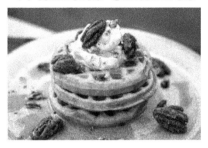

Preparation time: 20 minutes **Cooking time:** 15 minutes

Servings: 2

Ingredients:

- 2 tbsps. cream cheese
- ½ tsp. almonds flour
- ¼ tsp. baking powder
- 1 large egg
- ¼ cup chopped walnuts
- Pinch of stevia extract powder

Directions:

1. Preheat your waffle maker.
2. Spray waffle maker with cooking spray.
3. In a bowl, add cream cheese, almond flour, baking powder, egg, walnuts and stevia.
4. Mix all ingredients.

5. Spoon walnut batter in the waffle maker and cooking for about 2-3 minutes.
6. Let chaffles cool at room temperature before serving.

Nutrition:

Kcal 492, Fat: 36g, Net Carbs: 3g, Protein: 35g

Bacon Chaffles

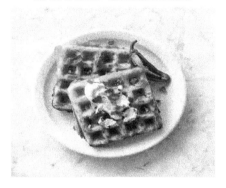

Preparation time: 20 minutes **Cooking time:** 15 minutes

Servings: 2

Ingredients:

- 1 egg
- ½ cup Swiss cheese
- 2 tablespoons cooked crumbled bacon

Directions:

1. Preheat your waffle maker.
2. Beat the egg in a bowl.
3. Stir in the cheese and bacon.
4. Pour half of the mixture into the device.
5. Close and cooking for 4 minutes.
6. Cooking the second chaffle using the same steps.

Nutrition:

Calories: 317 Total Fat: 18g Protein: 38g Total Carbs: 0g Fiber: 0g Net Carbs: 0g

Bacon Chaffles

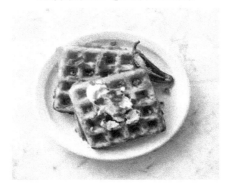

Preparation time: 20 minutes **Cooking time:** 15 minutes

Servings: 2

Ingredients:

- 1/4 cup heavy cream
- 4 oz. strawberry slice

Chaffle Ingredients:

- 1 egg
- ½ cup Mozzarella cheese

Directions:

1. Make 2 chaffles with chaffle ingredients.
2. Meanwhile, mix together cream and strawberries.
3. Spread this mixture over chaffle slice.

4. Drizzle chocolate sauce over a sandwich.

5. Serve and enjoy!

Nutrition:

Calories 369, Carbs 7 g, Fat 18 g, Protein 46 g, Sodium 811 mg, Sugar 0 g

Choco And Strawberries Chaffles

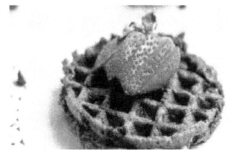

Preparation time: 10 minutes **Cooking time:** 5 minutes

Servings: 2

Ingredients:

- 1 tbsp. almond flour
- 1/2 cup strawberry puree
- 1/2 cup cheddar cheese
- 1 tbsp. cocoa powder
- ½ tsp. baking powder
- 1 large egg.
- 2 tbsps. coconut oil. melted
- 1/2 tsp. vanilla extract optional

Directions:

1. Preheat waffle iron while you are mixing the ingredients.

2. Melt oil in a microwave.

3. In a small mixing bowl, mix together flour, baking powder, flour, and vanilla until well combined.

4. Add egg, melted oil, ½ cup cheese and strawberry puree to the flour mixture.

5. Pour 1/8 cup cheese in a waffle maker and then pour the mixture in the center of greased waffle.

6. Again, sprinkle cheese on the batter.

7. Close the waffle maker.

8. Cooking chaffles for about 4-5 minutes until cooked and crispy.

9. Once chaffles are cooked, remove and enjoy!

Nutrition:

Calories 520, Carbs 3.7 g, Fat 24 g, Protein 67 g, Sodium 923 mg, Sugar 0 g

Coconut Flour Waffle

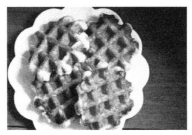

Preparation time: 5 minutes **Cooking time:** 5 minutes

Servings: 4

Ingredients:

- 8 eggs
- 1/2 cup of butter or coconut oil
- 1 tsp. of vanilla extract
- 1/2 tsp. salt
- 1/2 cup of coconut flour

Directions:

1. Pre heat the mini waffle maker.
2. Whisk the eggs in a bowl.
3. Then you add the melted butter or coconut oil, cinnamon, vanilla and salt, mix properly then you add the Coconut flour. Ensure the batter is thick.
4. Add the mixture into the mini waffle maker and allow

to cooking till it has a light brown appearance.

5. Serve with butter or maple syrup.

Nutrition:

Net Carbs: 6.8g; Calories: 357; Total Fat: 28.9g; Saturated Fat: 13.2g; Protein: 15.2g; Carbs: 8.9g; Fiber: 2.1g; Sugar: 3.9g

Easy Corn Dog Chaffle

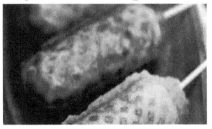

Preparation time: 15 minutes **Cooking time:** 5 minutes

Servings: 5

Ingredients:

- 2 eggs
- 1 cup Mexican cheese blend
- 1 tbs almond flour
- 1/2 tsp. cornbread extract
- 1/4 tsp. salt
- hot dogs with hot dog sticks

Directions:

1. Preheat corndog waffle maker.
2. In a small bowl, whip the eggs.
3. Add the remaining ingredients except the hotdogs.
4. Spray the corndog waffle maker with non-stick cooking spray. Fill the corndog waffle maker with the batter

halfway filled. Place a stick in the hot dog.

5. Place the hot dog in the batter and slightly press down.
6. Spread a small amount of better on top of the hot dog, just enough to fill it.
7. Makes about 4 to 5 chaffle corndogs.
8. Cooking the corndog chaffles for about 4 minutes or until golden brown.
9. When done, they will easily remove from the corndog waffle maker with a pair of tongs.
10. Serve with mustard, mayo, or sugar-free ketchup!

Nutrition:

Calories 304, Fat 8.3, Fiber 4.5, Carbs 1.6, Protein 7

Pecan Pie Cake Chaffle

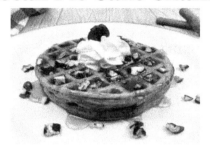

Preparation time: 15 minutes **Cooking time:** 5 minutes

Servings: 5

Ingredients:

For Pecan Pie Chaffle:

- Egg: 1
- Cream cheese: 2 tbsp.
- Maple extract: ½ tbsp.
- Almond flour: 4 tbsp.
- Sukrin Gold: 1 tbsp.
- Baking powder: ½ tbsp.
- Pecan: 2 tbsp. chopped
- Heavy whipping cream: 1 tbsp.

For Pecan Pie Filling:

- Butter: 2 tbsp.

- Sukrin Gold: 1 tbsp.
- Pecan: 2 tbsp. chopped
- Heavy whipping cream: 2 tbsp.
- Maple syrup: 2 tbsp.
- Egg yolk: 2 large
- Salt: a pinch

Directions:

1. In a small saucepan, add sweetener, butter, syrups, and heavy whipping cream and use a low flame to heat.
2. Mix all the ingredients well together.
3. Remove from heat and add egg yolks and mix.
4. Now put it on heat again and stir.
5. Add pecan and salt to the mixture and let it simmer.
6. It will thicken then remove from heat and let it rest.
7. For the chaffles, add all the ingredients except pecans and blend.
8. Now add pecan with a spoon.
9. Preheat a mini waffle maker if needed and grease it.
10. Pour the mixture to the lower plate of the waffle maker and spread it evenly to cover the plate properly and close the lid. Cooking for at least 4 minutes to get the desired crunch. Remove the chaffle from the heat and keep aside for around one minute 13.

11. Make as many chaffles as your mixture and waffle maker allow 14. Add 1/3 the previously prepared pecan pie filling to the chaffle and arrange like a cake.

Nutrition:

Calories: 205 Fat: 2 g Protein: 13 g Carbs: 31 g Fiber: 17g

Banana Cake Pudding Chaffle

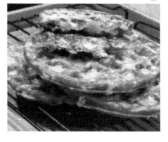

Preparation time: 15 minutes **Cooking time:** 1hr

Servings: 2

Ingredients:

For Banana Chaffle:

- Cream cheese: 2 tbsp.
- Banana extract: 1 tsp.
- Mozzarella cheese: ¼ cup
- Egg: 1
- Sweetener: 2 tbsp.
- Almond flour: 4 tbsp.
- Baking powder: 1 tsp.

For Banana Pudding:

- Egg yolk: 1 large
- Powdered sweetener: 3 tbsp.

- Xanthan gum: ½ tsp.
- Heavy whipping cream: 1/2 cup
- Banana extract: ½ tsp.
- Salt: a pinch

Directions:

1. In a pan, add powdered sweetener, heavy cream, and egg yolk and whisk continuously so the mixture thickens.
2. Simmer for a minute only.
3. Add xanthan gum to the mixture and whisk again.
4. Remove the pan from heat and add banana extract and salt and mix them all well.
5. Shift the mixture to a glass dish and refrigerate the pudding. Preheat a mini waffle maker if needed and grease it.
6. In a mixing bowl, add all the chaffle ingredients.
7. Mix them all well and pour the mixture to the lower plate of the waffle maker.
8. Close the lid.
9. Cooking for at least 5 minutes to get the desired crunch. Remove the chaffle from the heat and keep aside for around a few minutes.
10. Stack chaffles and pudding one by one to form a cake.

Nutrition:

Calories 187 Fat 16.7 g Saturated fat 4.1 g Carbohydrates 6.7 g
Fiber 2 g Protein 3.3 g

Chaffle Churros

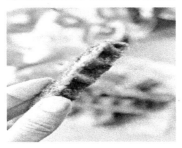

Preparation time: 15 minutes **Cooking time:** 5 minutes

Servings: 2

Ingredients:

- 1 Tbsp. almond flour

- ½ tsp. vanilla extract
- 1 tsp. cinnamon, divided
- ¼ tsp. baking powder
- ½ cup shredded mozzarella
- 1 Tbsp. swerve confectioners' sugar substitute
- 1 Tbsp. swerve brown sugar substitute
- 1 Tbsp. butter, melted
- 1 egg

Directions:

1. Turn on waffle maker to heat and oil it with cooking

spray. Mix egg, flour, vanilla extract, ½ tsp. cinnamon, baking powder, mozzarella, and sugar substitute in a bowl.

2. Place half of the mixture into waffle maker and cooking for 3-5 minutes, or until desired doneness. Remove and place the second half of the batter into the maker.
3. Cut chaffles into strips. 5. Place strips in a bowl and cover with melted butter.
4. Mix brown sugar substitute and the remaining cinnamon in a bowl. Pour sugar mixture over the strips and toss to coat them well.

Nutrition:

Calories: 372, Fat: 16g, Carbs: 3g, Protein: 40g

Fluffy Keto Chaffle

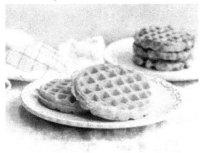

Preparation time: 5 minutes **Cooking time:** 5 minutes

Servings: 1

Ingredients:

- 1 egg
- 1/2 cup cheddar cheese, shredded

Directions:

1. Switch on the waffle maker according to manufacturer's Directions.
2. Crack egg and combine with cheddar cheese in a small bowl. Place half batter on waffle maker and spread evenly.
3. Cooking for 4 minutes or until as desired.
4. Gently remove from waffle maker and set aside for 2 minutes so it cools down and become crispy.

5. Repeat for remaining batter.
6. Serve with desired toppings

Nutrition:

Calories 92, Fat 1.4, Fiber 0.2, Carbs 1.5, Protein 17.4

Crispy Sandwich Chaffle

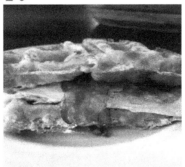

Preparation time: 5 minutes **Cooking time:** 5 minutes

Servings: 1

Ingredients:

- 1egg
- 1/2 cup cheddar cheese, shredded
- 1 tbsp. coconut flour

Directions:

1. Using a mini waffle maker, preheat according to maker's Directions. Combine egg and cheddar cheese in a mixing bowl. Stir thoroughly.
2. Add coconut flour for added texture if so desired.
3. Place half batter on waffle maker and spread evenly.
4. Cooking for 4 minutes or until as desired.
5. Gently remove from waffle maker and set aside for 2

minutes so it cools down and become crispy. Repeat for remaining batter.

6. Stuff 2 chaffles with desired sandwich.

Nutrition:

Calories: 472 Carbohydrates: 1.2 Protein: 32.6 Fat: 42.4 Sugar: 0 Fiber: 0.4

Jalapeno Bacon Swiss Chaffle

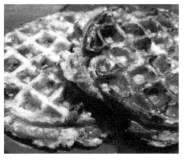

Preparation time: 5 minutes **Cooking time:** 5 minutes

Servings: 1

Ingredients:

- Shredded Swiss cheese: ½ cup
- Fresh jalapenos: 1 tablespoon
- Bacon piece: 2 tablespoons
- Egg: 1

Directions:

1. First, preheat and grease the waffle maker.
2. Using a pan, cooking the bacon pieces, put off the heat and shred the cheese and egg.
3. Add in the diced fresh jalapenos and mix evenly.
4. Heat the waffle makers to get the mixture into a crispy form. Repeat the process for the remaining mixture.

5. Serve the dish to enjoy.

Nutrition:

Calories 329, Fat 16, Carbs 10, Protein 23

Chaffle & Egg Sandwich

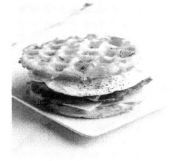

Preparation time: 5 minutes **Cooking time:** 15 minutes

Servings: 2

Ingredients:

- 2 Mini keto chaffle
- 2 slice cheddar cheese
- 1 egg simple omelet

Directions:

1. Preheat your oven on 4000 F.
2. Arrange egg omelet and cheese slice between chaffles.
3. Bake in the preheated oven for about 4-5 minutes until cheese is melted. Once the cheese is melted, remove from the oven.
4. Serve and enjoy!

Nutrition:

Calories 224 Carb 8g Fat 16g Cholesterol 90mg Sodium 527mg Fiber 2g Protein 10g Sugar 2g

Burger Chaffle

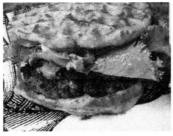

Preparation time: 5 minutes **Cooking time:** 15 minutes

Servings: 2

Ingredients:

For the Cheeseburgers:

- 1/3 lb. beef, ground
- ½ tsp garlic salt
- 3 slices American cheese

For the Chaffles:

- 1 large egg
- ½ cup mozzarella, finely shredded
- Salt and ground pepper to taste

For the Big Mac Sauce:

- 2 tsp mayonnaise

- 1 tsp ketchup

To Assemble:

- 2 tbsp lettuce, shredded
- 4 dill pickles
- 2 tsp onion, minced

Directions:

1. Take your burger patties and place them on one chaffle. Top with shredded lettuce, onions and pickles.
2. Spread the sauce over the other chaffle and place it on top of the veggies, sauce side down.

Nutrition:

Calories: 298, Fat: 17g, Carbs: 7.2, Protein: 23g

Ham Chaffle

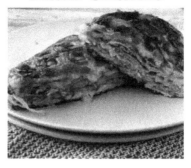

Preparation time: 10 minutes **Cooking time:** 15 minutes

Servings: 2

Ingredients:

- 2 large organic eggs
- 6 tablespoons butter, melted
- 2 scoops unflavored whey protein powder
- 1 teaspoon organic baking powder
- Salt, to taste
- 1-ounce sugar-free ham, chopped finely
- 1-ounce Cheddar cheese, shredded
- 1/8 teaspoon paprika

Directions:

1. Preheat a waffle iron and then grease it.
2. In a bowl place egg yolk, butter, protein powder, baking

powder and salt and beat until well combined.

3. Add the ham steak pieces, cheese and paprika and stir to combine.

4. In another bowl, place 2 egg whites and a pinch of salt and with an electric hand mixer and beat until stiff peaks form. Gently fold the whipped egg whites into the egg yolk mixture in 2 batches.

5. Place ¼ of the mixture into preheated waffle iron and cook for about 3-4 minutes or until golden brown.

6. Repeat with the remaining mixture.

7. Serve warm.

Nutrition:

Net Carbs: 2.4g; Calories: 321; Total Fat: 21.4g; Saturated Fat: 10.6g; Protein: 27.3g; Carbs: 4.8g; Fiber: 2.4g; Sugar: 1.2g

Garlic and Spinach Chaffles

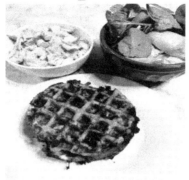

Preparation time: 10 minutes **Cooking time:** 5 minutes

Servings: 2

Ingredients:

- 1 cup egg whites
- 1 tsp. Italian spice
- 2 tsps. coconut flour
- ½ tsp. Vanilla
- 1 tsp. baking powder
- 1 tsp. baking soda
- 1 cup mozzarella cheese, grated
- 1/2 tsp. garlic powder
- 1 cup chopped spinach

Directions:

1. Switch on your square waffle maker. Spray with non-stick spray.
2. Beat egg whites with beater, until fluffy and white.
3. Add pumpkin puree, pumpkin pie spice, coconut flour in egg whites and beat again.
4. Stir in the cheese, powder, garlic powder, baking soda, and powder.
5. Sprinkle chopped spinach on a waffle maker.
6. Pour the batter in waffle maker over chopped spinach.
7. Close the maker and cook for about 4-5 minutes Utes.
8. Remove chaffles from the maker.
9. Serve hot and enjoy!

Nutrition:

Net Carbs: 3.5g; Calories: 202.5; Total Fat: 24.2g; Saturated Fat: 6g; Protein: 22.7g; Carbs: 4g; Fiber: 0.5g; Sugar: 1.1g

Italian Bread Chaffle

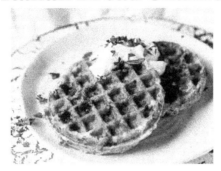

Preparation time: 15 minutes **Cooking time:** 25 minutes

Servings: 2

Ingredients:

For the Chaffle:

- Egg: 2
- Mozzarella cheese: 1 cup (shredded)
- Garlic powder: ½ tsp.
- Italian seasoning: 1 tsp.
- Cream cheese: 1 tsp.

For the Garlic Butter Topping:

- Garlic powder: ½ tsp.
- Italian seasoning: ½ tsp.
- Butter: 1 tbsp.

For Cheesy Bread:

- Mozzarella cheese: 2 tbsp. (shredded)
- Parsley: 1 tbsp

Directions:

1. Preheat a mini waffle maker if needed and grease it.
2. In a mixing bowl, add all the ingredients of the chaffle and mix well.
3. Pour the mixture to the lower plate of the waffle maker and spread it evenly to cover the plate properly and close the lid.
4. Cooking for at least 4 minutes to get the desired crunch.
5. In the meanwhile, melt butter and add the garlic butter ingredients.
6. Remove the chaffle from the heat and apply the garlic butter immediately. Make as many chaffles as your mixture and waffle maker allow.
7. Put the chaffles on the baking tray and sprinkle the Mozzarella cheese on the chaffles.
8. Bake for 5 minutes in an oven at 350 degrees to melt the cheese.
9. Serve hot and enjoy.

Nutrition:

Calories: 181; Total Fat: 19g; Carbs: 4g; Net Carbs: 2g; Fiber: 2g; Protein: 1g

Coconut Chaffle

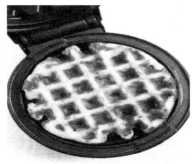

Preparation time: 10 minutes **Cooking time:** 5 minutes

Servings: 2

Ingredients:

- 1 egg
- 1 oz. cream cheese,
- 1 oz. cheddar cheese
- 2 tbsps. coconut flour
- 1 tsp. stevia
- 1 tbsp. coconut oil, melted
- 1/2 tsp. coconut extract
- 2 eggs, soft boil for serving

Directions:

1. Heat your waffle maker and grease with cooking spray.
2. Mix together all chaffles ingredients in a bowl.

3. Pour chaffle batter in a preheated waffle maker.
4. Close the lid.
5. Cooking chaffles for about 2-3 minutes until golden brown. Serve with boil egg and enjoy.

Nutrition:

Calories: 331 kcal Protein: 11.84 g Fat: 30.92 g Carbohydrates: 1.06g

Beef Meatballs on A Chaffle

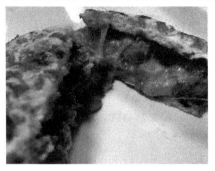

Preparation time: 10 minutes **Cooking time:** 25 minutes

Servings: 4

Ingredients:

- Batter
- 4 eggs
- 2½ cups grated gouda cheese
- ¼ cup heavy cream
- Salt and pepper to taste
- 1 spring onion, finely chopped Beef meatballs
- 1 pound ground beef S
- alt and pepper to taste
- 2 teaspoons Dijon mustard
- 1 spring onion, finely chopped
- 5 tablespoons almond flour

- 2 tablespoons butter
- 2 tablespoons cooking spray to brush the waffle maker
- 2 tablespoons freshly chopped parsley

Directions:

1. Preheat the waffle maker.
2. Add the eggs, grated gouda cheese, heavy cream, salt and pepper and finely chopped spring onion to a bowl.
3. Mix until combined and batter forms.
4. Brush the heated waffle maker with cooking spray and add a few tablespoons of the batter.
5. Close the lid and cooking for about 7 minutes depending on your waffle maker.
6. Meanwhile, mix the ground beef meat, salt and pepper, Dijon mustard, chopped spring onion and almond flour in a large bowl.
7. Form small meatballs with your hands.
8. Heat the butter in a nonstick frying pan and cooking the beef meatballs for about 3-4 minutes on each side.
9. Serve each chaffle with a couple of meatballs and some freshly chopped parsley on top.

Nutrition:

Calories 200, Fat 2, Fiber 3, Carbs 7, Protein 5

Ricotta Chaffle

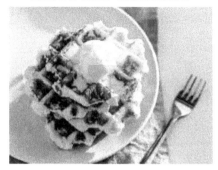

Preparation time: 10 minutes **Cooking time:** 10 minutes

Servings: 4

Ingredients:

- 2 cups coconut flour
- 1 and ½ cups coconut milk
- 2 tablespoons olive oil
- A pinch of salt and black pepper
- ½ cup ricotta cheese
- 1 teaspoon baking powder
- 2 eggs, whisked
- ½ cup chives, chopped
- 1 red chili pepper, minced
- 1 jalapeno, choppe

Directions:

1. In a bowl, mix the flour with the milk, oil and the other ingredients and whisk well.
2. Heat up the waffle iron, pour ¼ of the batter, cooking for 10 minutes and transfer to a plate.
3. Repeat with the rest of the chaffle mix and serve.

Nutrition:

Net Carbs: 0.8g; Calories: 737.6; Total Fat: 72.1g; Saturated Fat: 8.6g; Protein: 20.2g; Carbs: 1.8g; Fiber: 0.6g; Sugar: 1g

Creamy Pistachios Chaffles

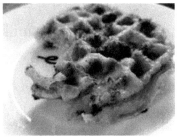

Preparation time: 5 minutes **Cooking time:** 10 minutes

Servings: 2

Ingredients:

- Egg: 1
- Mozzarella cheese: ½ cup shredded
- Swerve/Monkfruit: 1 tsp.
- Vanilla extract: 1/2 tsp.
- Coconut flour: 1 tbsp.
- Cream: ¼ cup
- Pistachios: ½ cup chopped

Directions:

1. Add all the chaffle ingredients in a bowl and whisk.
2. Preheat your mini waffle iron if needed and grease it.
3. Cooking your mixture in the mini waffle iron for at least 4 minutes.

4. Make as many chaffles as you can and spread cream or low-carb ice cream on top.

Nutrition:

Calories 220, Fat 8, Fiber 10, Carbs 36, Protein 10

Parmesan Chaffles

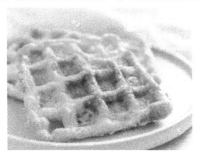

Preparation time: 5 minutes **Cooking time:** 5 minutes

Servings: 2

Ingredients:

- 1 Tbsp fresh garlic minced
- 2 Tbsp butter
- 1-oz cream cheese, cubed
- 2 Tbsp almond flour
- 1 tsp baking soda
- 2 large eggs
- 1 tsp dried chives
- ½ cup parmesan cheese, shredded
- ¾ cup mozzarella cheese, shredded

Directions:

1. Heat cream cheese and butter in a saucepan over

medium-low until melted.

2. Add garlic and cook, stirring, for minutes.

3. Turn on waffle maker to heat and oil it with cooking spray.

4. In a small mixing bowl, whisk together flour and baking soda, then set aside.

5. In a separate bowl, beat eggs for 1 minute 30 seconds on high, then add in cream cheese mixture and beat for 60 seconds more.

6. Add flour mixture, chives, and cheeses to the bowl and stir well.

7. Add ¼ cup batter to waffle maker.

8. Close and cook for 4 minutes, until golden brown.

9. Repeat for remaining batter.

10. Add favorite toppings and serve.

Nutrition:

Calories: 236 Total Fat: 23g Protein: 6g Total Carbs: 5g Fiber: 3g Net Carbs: 2g Cholesterol: 0mg

Chaffles With Berries

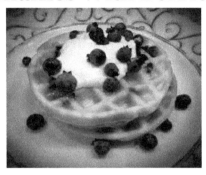

Preparation time: 10 minutes **Cooking time:** 25 minutes

Servings: 4

Ingredients:

- 1cup egg whites
- 1 cup cheddar cheese, shredded
- ¼ cup almond flour
- ¼ cup heavy cream

Topping

- 4 oz. raspberries
- 4 oz. strawberries.
- 1 oz. keto chocolate flakes
- 1 oz. feta cheese.

Directions:

1. Preheat your square waffle maker and grease with cooking spray.
2. Beat egg white in a small bowl with flour.
3. Add shredded cheese to the egg whites and flour mixture and mix well.
4. Add cream and cheese to the egg mixture.
5. Pour Chaffles batter in a waffle maker and close the lid.
6. Cook chaffles for about 4 minutes Utes until crispy and brown.
7. Carefully remove chaffles from the maker.
8. Serve with berries, cheese, and chocolate on top.

Nutrition:

Protein: 28% 68 kcal Fat: 67% 163 kcal Carbohydrates: 5% 12 kcal

Vanilla Berries

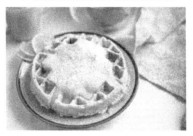

Preparation time: 10 minutes **Cooking time:** 25 minutes

Servings: 4

Ingredients:

- 1 egg, beaten
- ½ cup finely grated mozzarella cheese
- 1 tbsp cream cheese, softened
- 1 tbsp sugar-free maple syrup
- 2 strawberries, sliced
- 2 raspberries, slices
- ¼ tsp blackberry extract
- ¼ tsp vanilla extract
- ½ cup plain yogurt for serving

Directions:

1. Preheat the waffle iron.
2. In a medium bowl, mix all the ingredients except the

yogurt. Open the iron, lightly grease with cooking spray and pour in a quarter of the mixture.

3. Close the iron and cook until golden brown and crispy, 7 minutes.
4. Remove the chaffle onto a plate and set aside.
5. Make three more chaffles with the remaining mixture.
6. To serve: top with the yogurt and enjoy.

Nutrition:

Calories: 99 Cal Total Fat: 8 g Saturated Fat: 0 g Cholesterol: 0 mg Sodium: 0 mg Total Carbs: 4 g 30

Chicken Quesadilla Chaffle

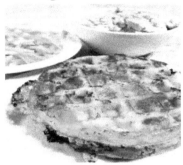

Preparation time: 10 minutes **Cooking time:** 15 minutes

Servings: 2

Ingredients:

- 1 egg, beaten
- ¼ tsp taco seasoning
- 1/3 cup finely grated cheddar cheese
- 1/3 cup cooked chopped chicken

Directions:

1. Preheat the waffle iron.
2. In a medium bowl, mix the eggs, taco seasoning, and cheddar cheese. Add the chicken and combine well.
3. Open the iron, lightly grease with cooking spray and pour in half of the mixture.
4. Close the iron and cook until brown and crispy, 7

minutes. Remove the chaffle onto a plate and set aside.

5. Make another chaffle using the remaining mixture.
6. Serve afterward.

Nutrition:

Calories: 99 Cal Total Fat: 8 g Saturated Fat: 0 g Cholesterol: 0 mg Sodium: 0 mg Total Carbs: 4 g

Cinnamon Swirls Chaffle

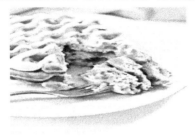

Preparation time: 10 minutes **Cooking time:** 5 minutes

Servings: 2

Ingredients:

Icing

- Butter: 2 tablespoons unsalted butter
- Cream cheese: 2 oz. softened
- Vanilla: 1 teaspoon
- Splenda: 2 tablespoons

Chaffle

- Egg: 2
- Almond flour: 2 tablespoons
- Cinnamon: 2 teaspoons
- Splenda: 2 tablespoons
- Cream Cheese: 2 oz. softened

- Vanilla Extract: 2 teaspoons Vanilla extract: 2 teaspoons

Cinnamon Drizzle

- Splenda: 2 tablespoons
- Cinnamon: 2 teaspoons
- Butter: 1 tablespoon

Directions:

1. Preheat and grease a waffle maker a combined mixture of all ingredients, evenly mixed and pour into the waffle maker.
2. Cooking for 4 minutes till chaffles turns crispy, and then set aside.
3. Using a mixing bowl, a mix of all ingredients for icing and the cinnamon drizzle, then heat using a microwave for 12 seconds to soften.
4. Pour heated icing and cinnamon on the cool chaffles to enjoy.

Nutrition:

Calories 134 Kcal Fat: 13.1 g Protein: 2.2 g Net carb: 1.1 g

Chaffles With Sausage

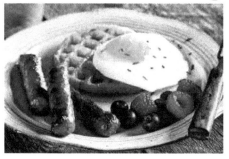

Preparation time: 5 minutes **Cooking time:** 15 minutes

Servings: 2

Ingredients:

- 1/2 cup cheddar cheese
- 1/2 tsp. baking powder
- 1/4 cup egg whites
- 2 tsp. pumpkin spice
- 1 egg, whole
- 2 chicken sausage
- 2 slice bacon
- salt and pepper to taste
- 1 tsp. avocado oil

Directions:

1. Mix together all ingredients in a bowl.

2. Allow batter to sit while waffle iron warms.

3. Spray waffle iron with nonstick spray.

4. Pour batter in the waffle maker and cooking according to the directions of the manufacturer.

5. Meanwhile, heat oil in a pan and fry the egg, according to your choice and transfer it to a plate.

6. In the same pan, fry bacon slice and sausage on medium heat for about 2-3 minutes until cooked.

7. Once chaffles are cooked thoroughly, remove them from the maker.

8. Serve with fried egg, bacon slice, sausages and enjoy!

Nutrition:

Calories: 319 Fat: 24 g Net Carbohydrates: 1 g Protein: 25 g

CPSIA information can be obtained
at www.ICGtesting.com
Printed in the USA
BVHW011429170321
602756BV00001B/20